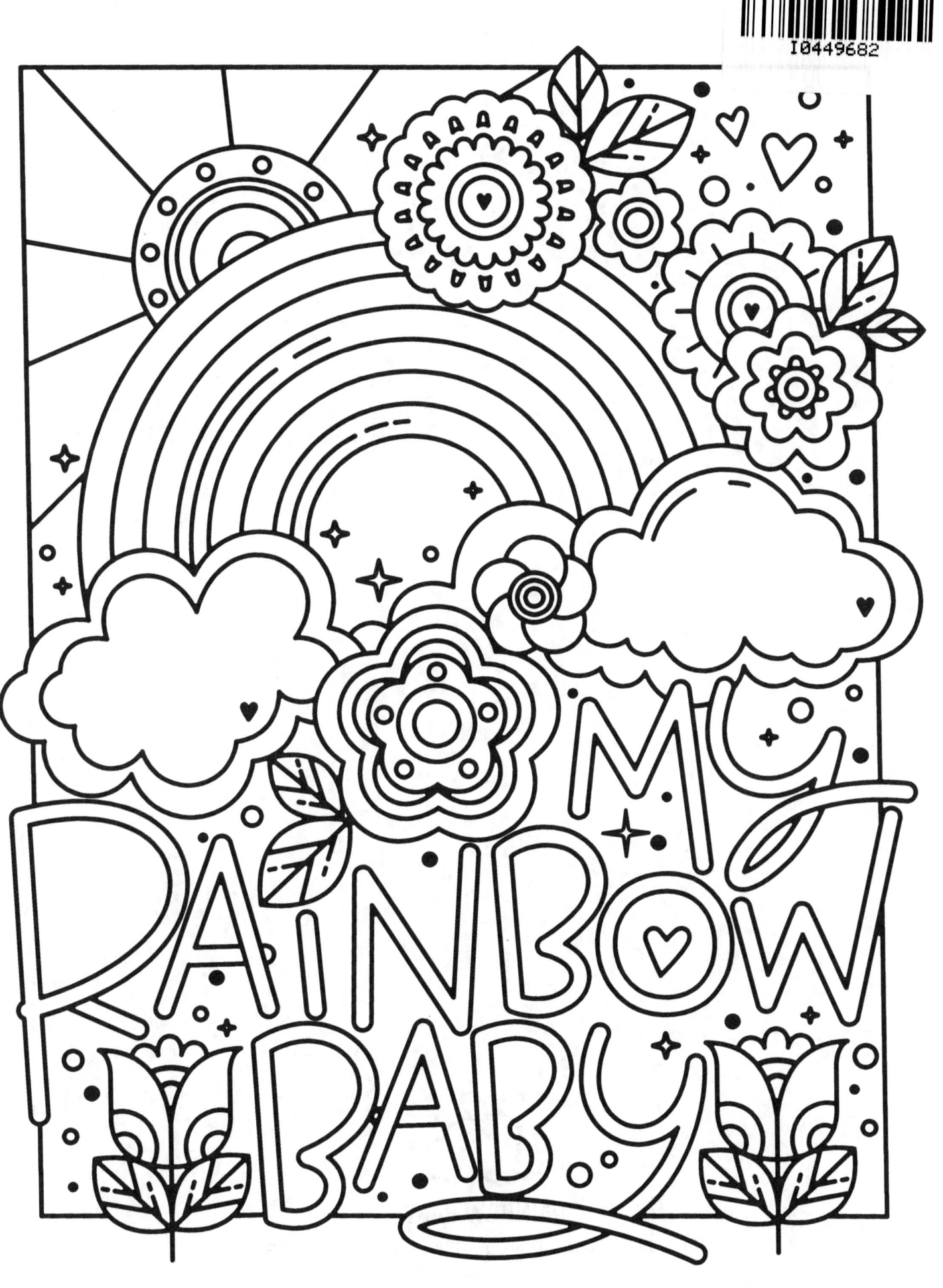

RAINBOW BABY
This rain is going to stop. the sun will soon shine.

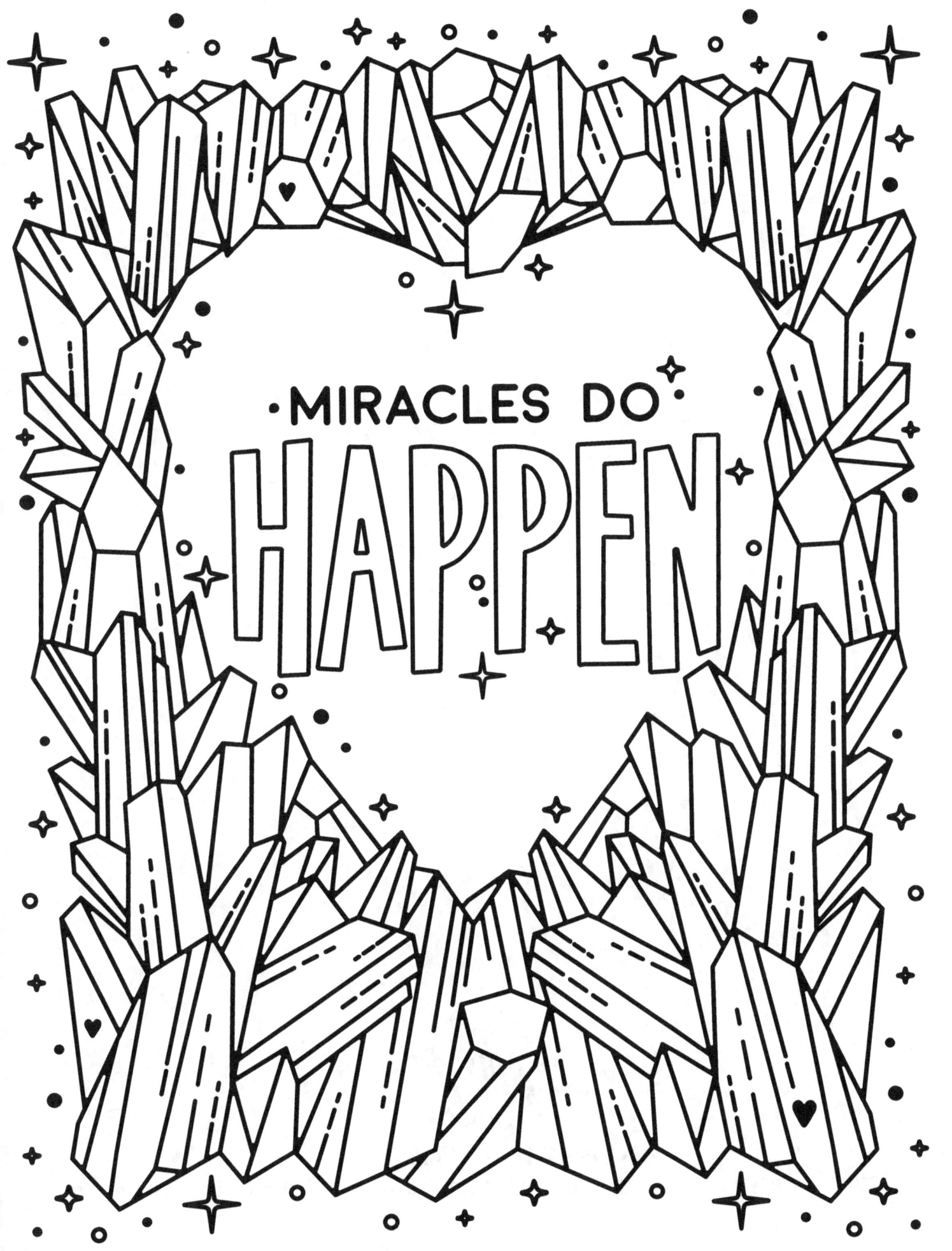

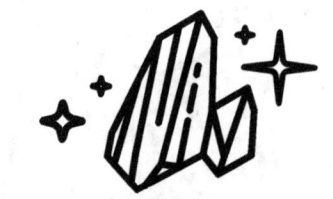

MIRACLES DO HAPPEN

Our story will be a great book with these words on the last page "and they lived happily ever after"

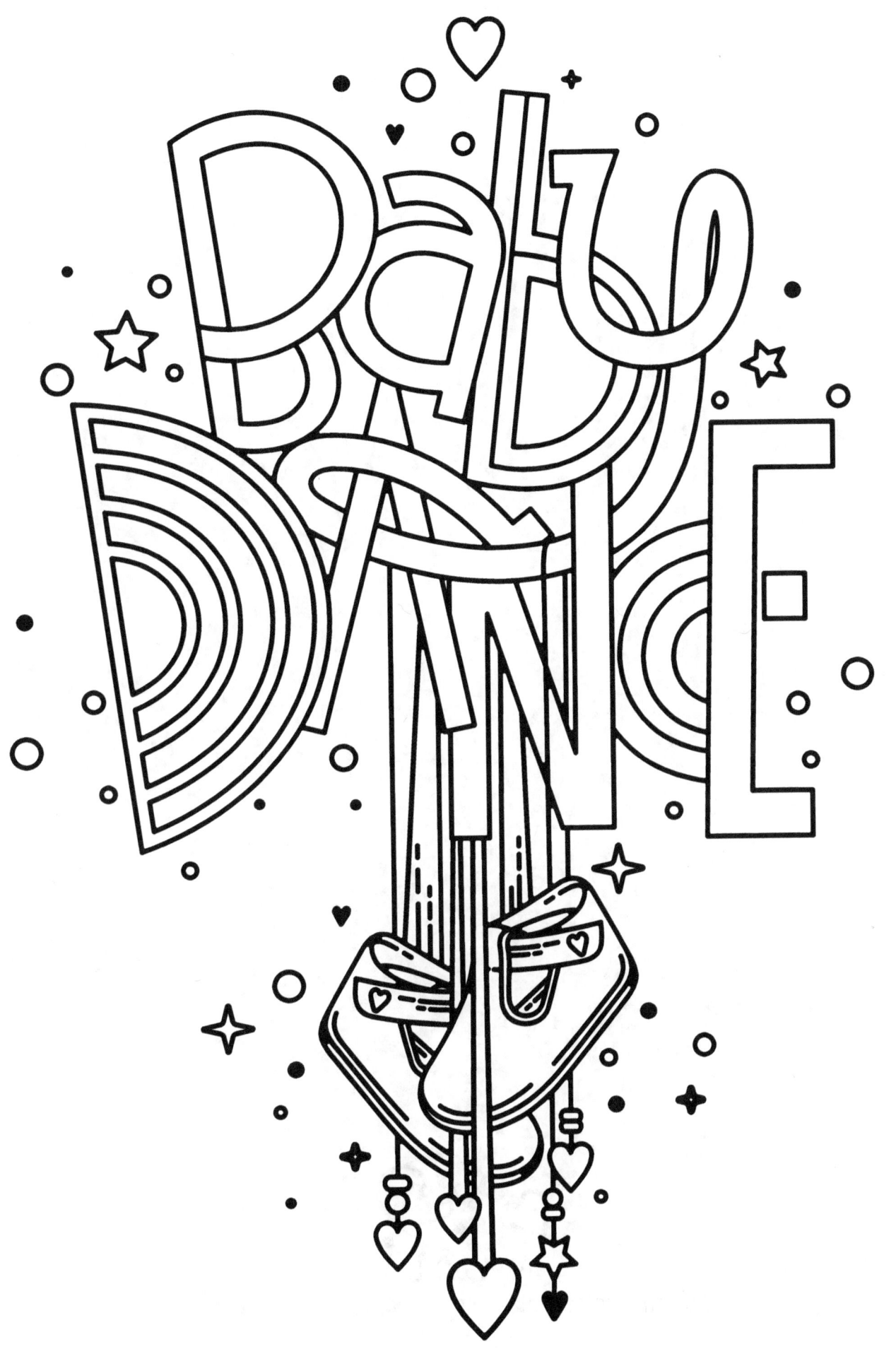

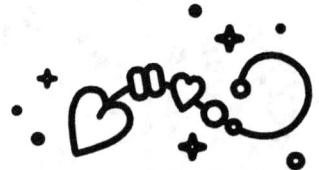

BABY DANCE

We can touch the stars. And we will bring one back.

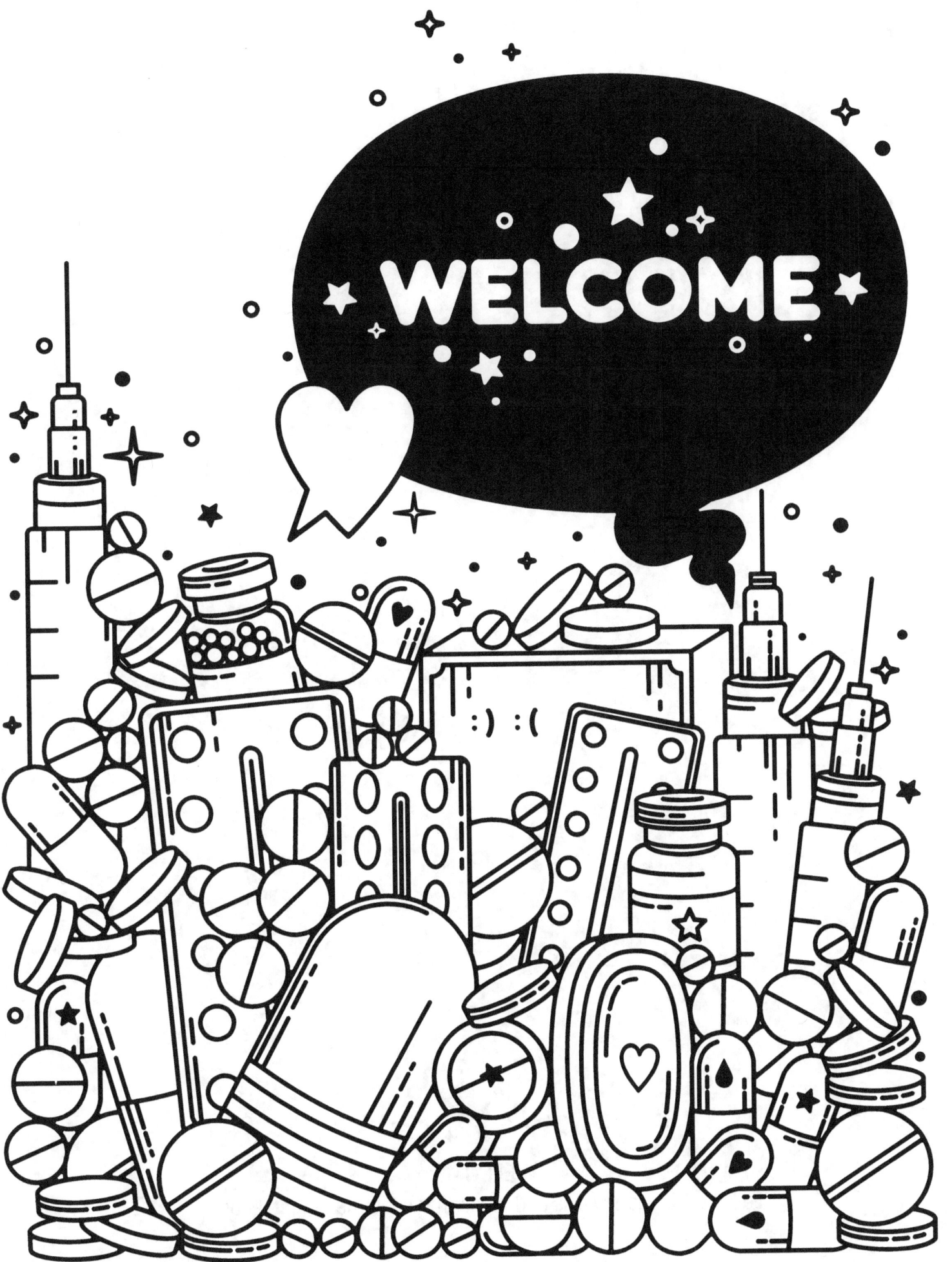

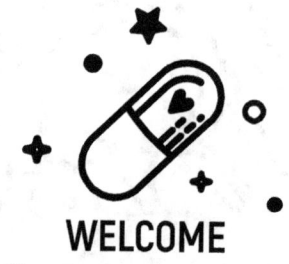

WELCOME

Let's be friends, my pills and meds. You keep me alright. Peace.

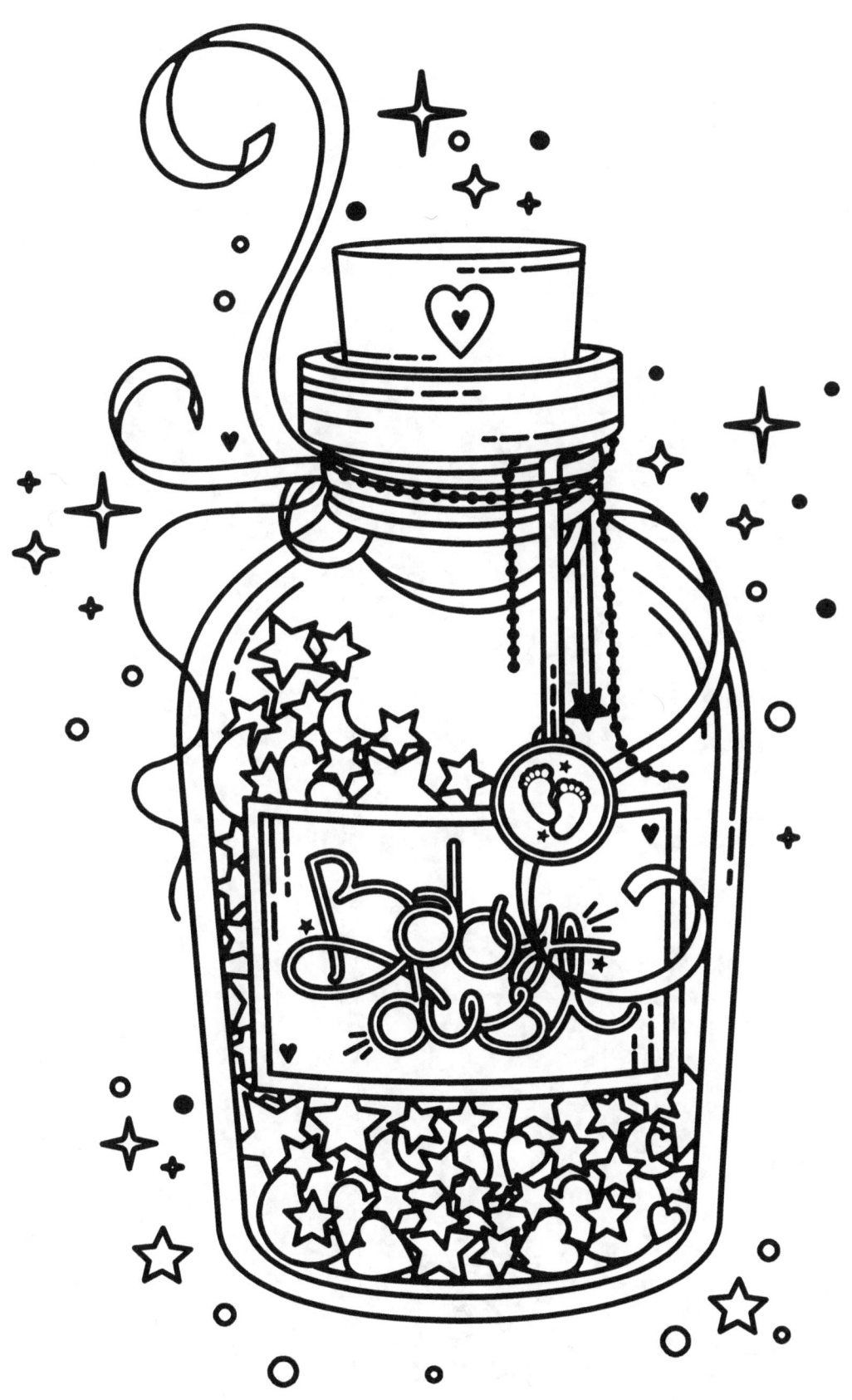

· BABY DUST ·

We are so lucky already. We are magic.

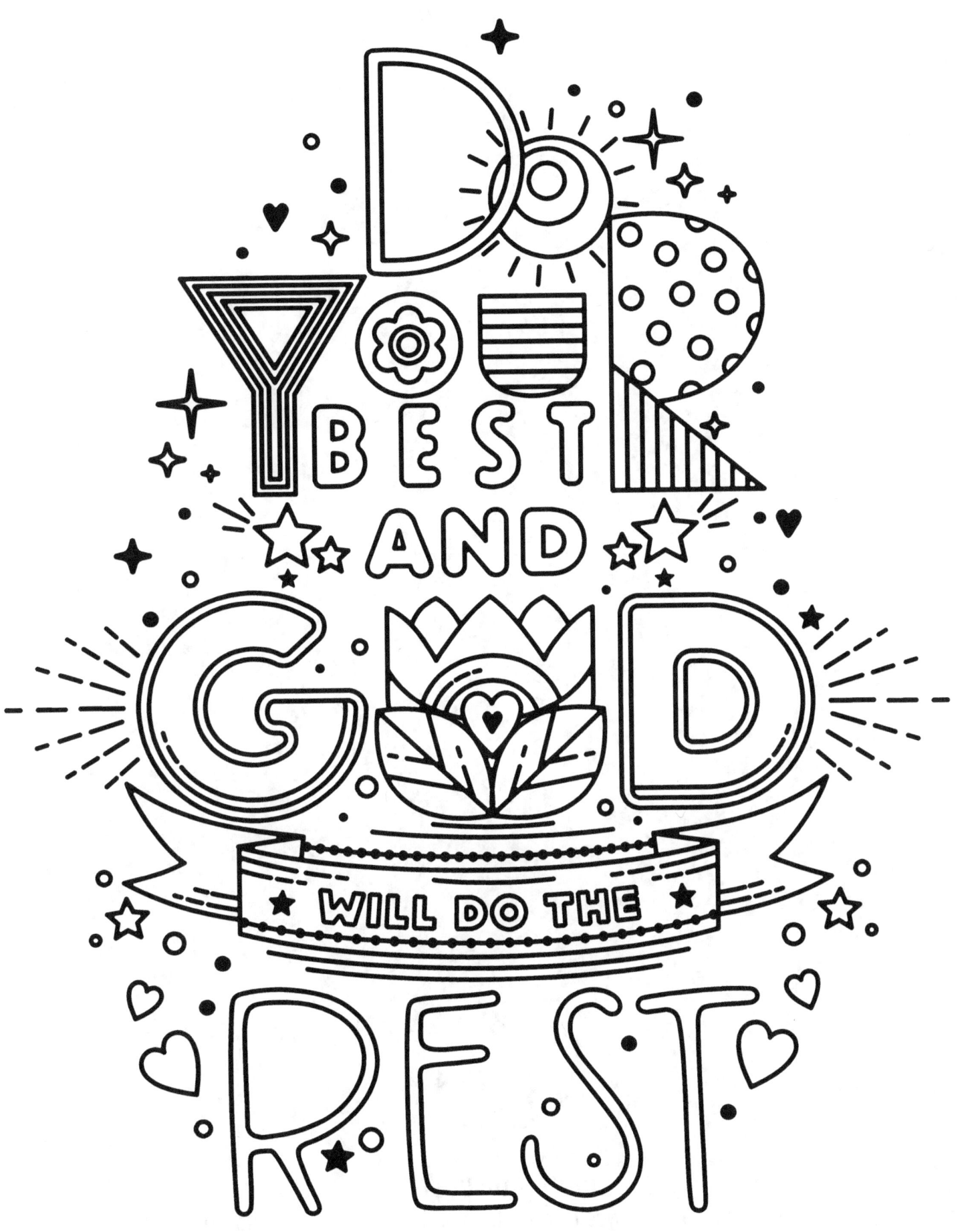

DO YOUR BEST AND GOD WILL DO THE REST

DO YOUR BEST
I take great care of myself. I eat, sleep and think my best all day long.

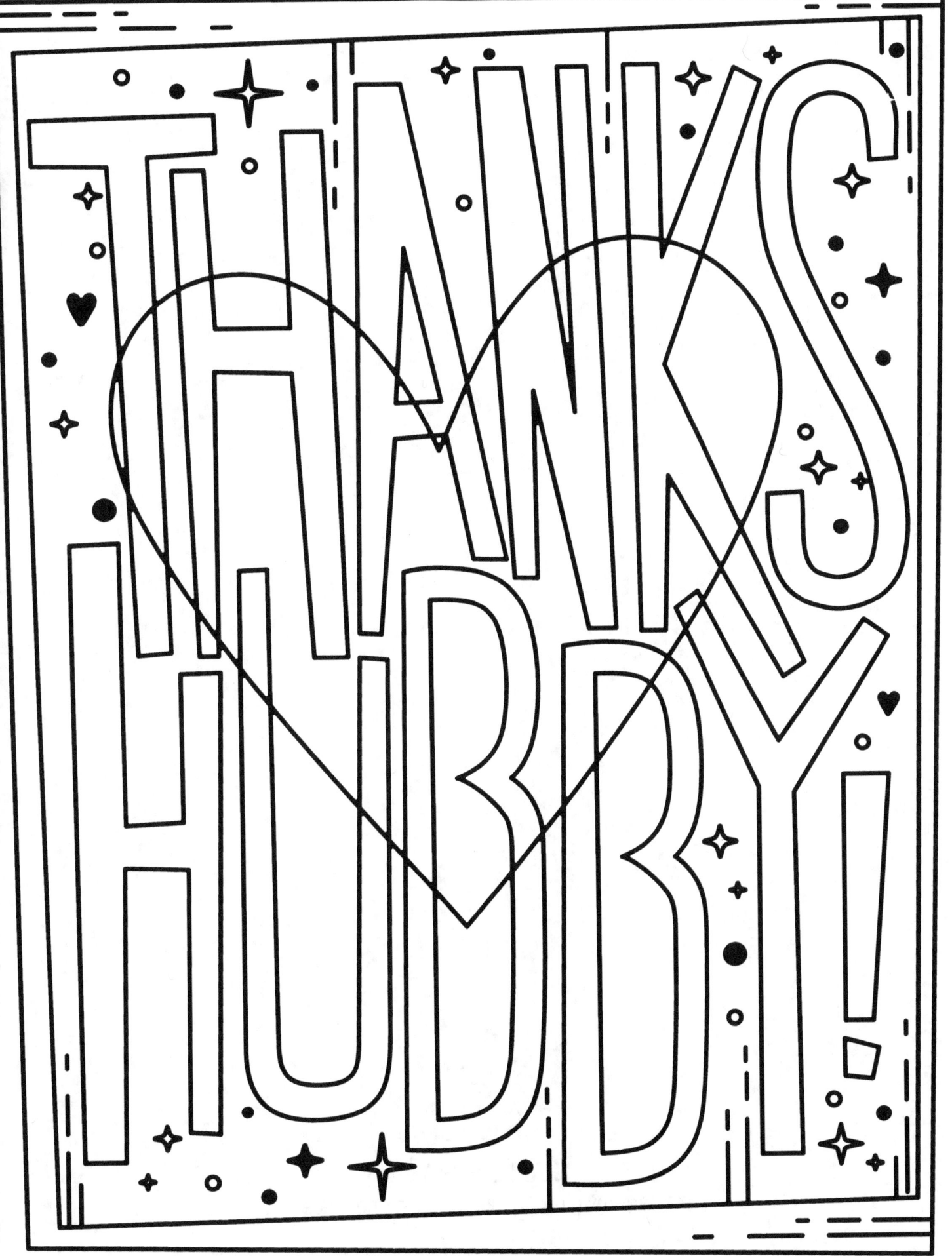

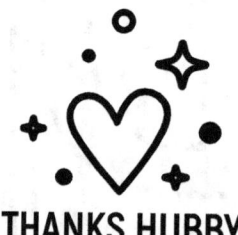

THANKS HUBBY

You are my glue. You keep me in one piece.

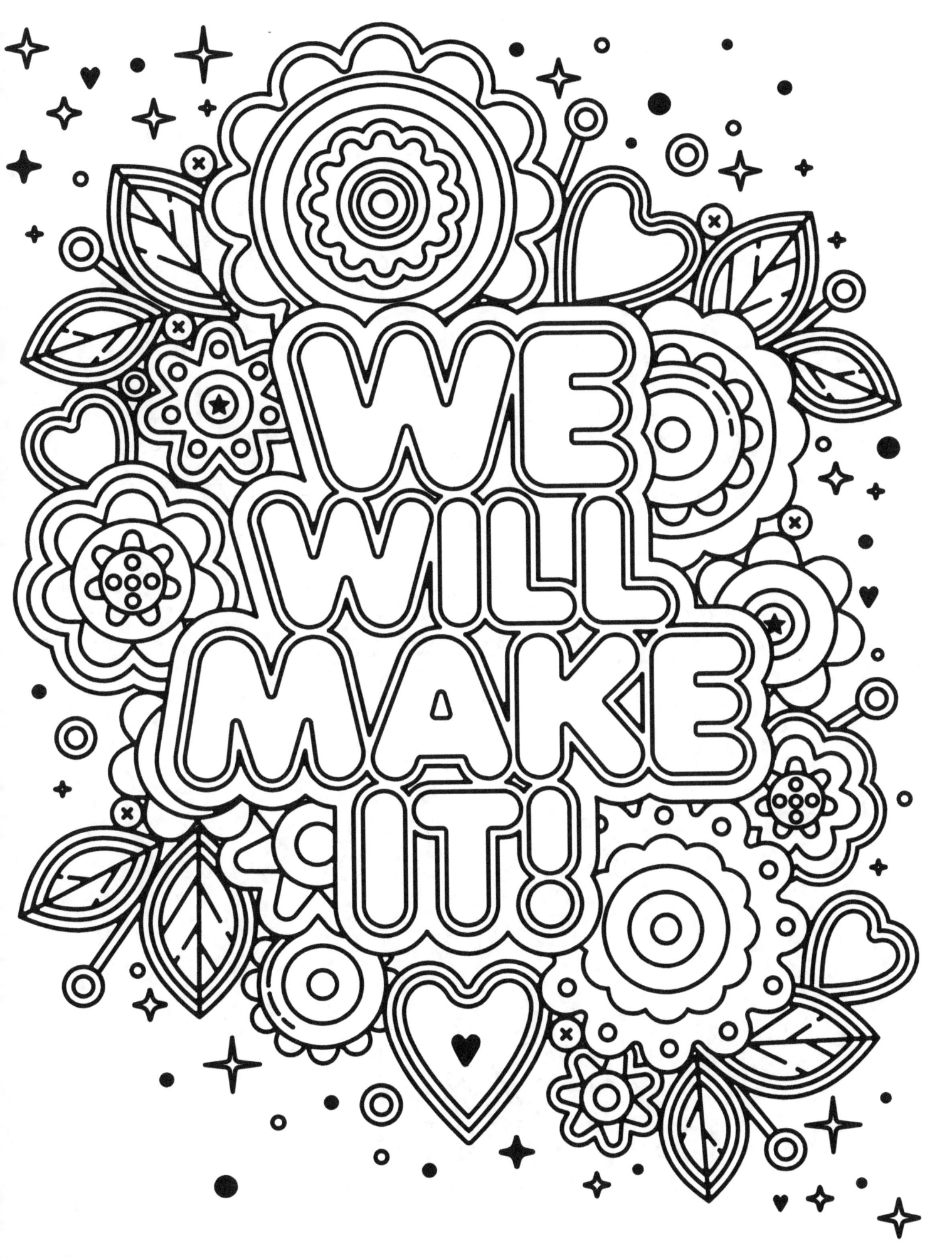

WE WILL MAKE IT
In this ride, I love my seat beside you..

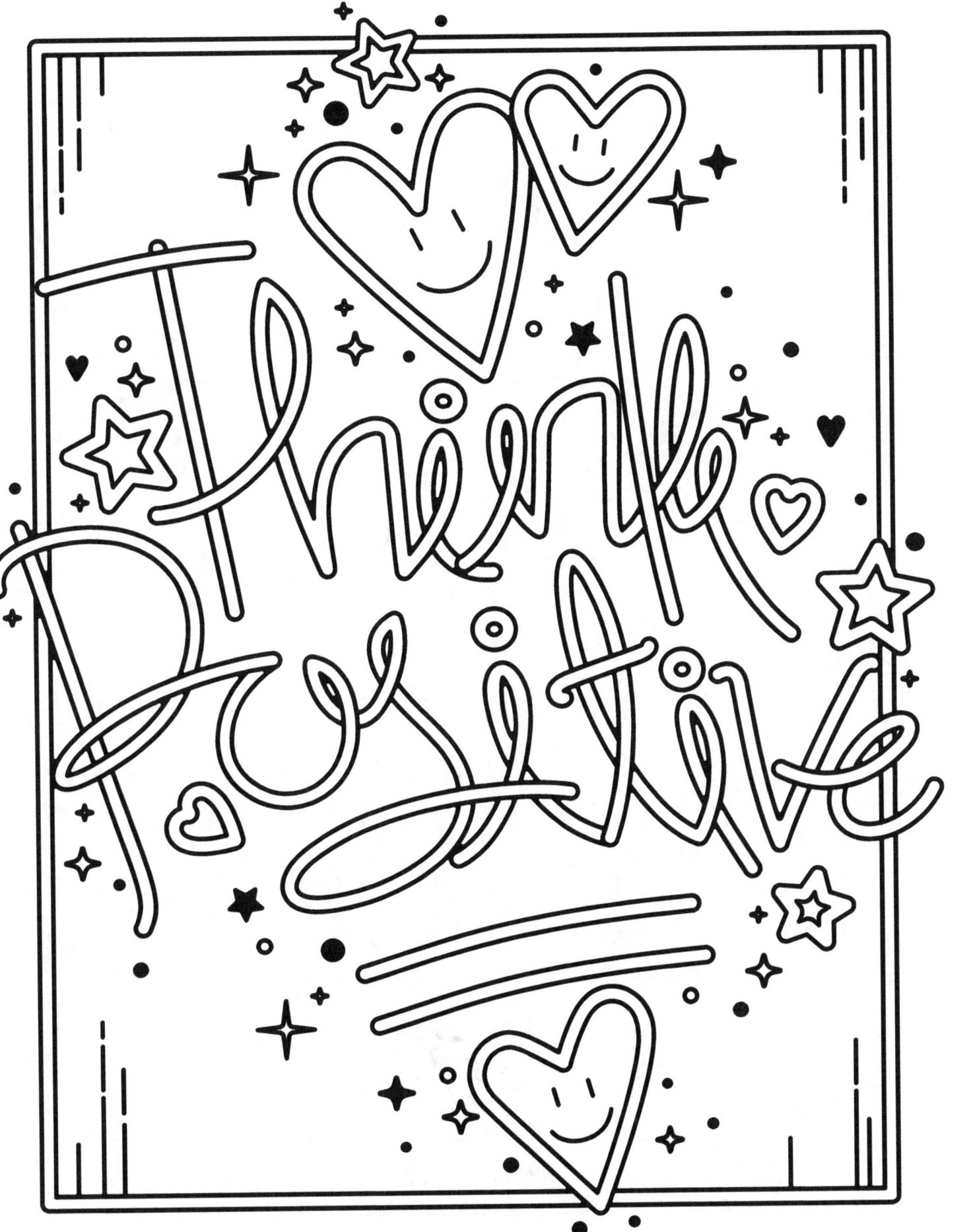

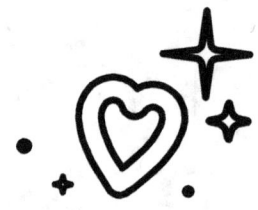

THINK POSITIVE
I take control of my thoughts. My mind is happy and optimistic.

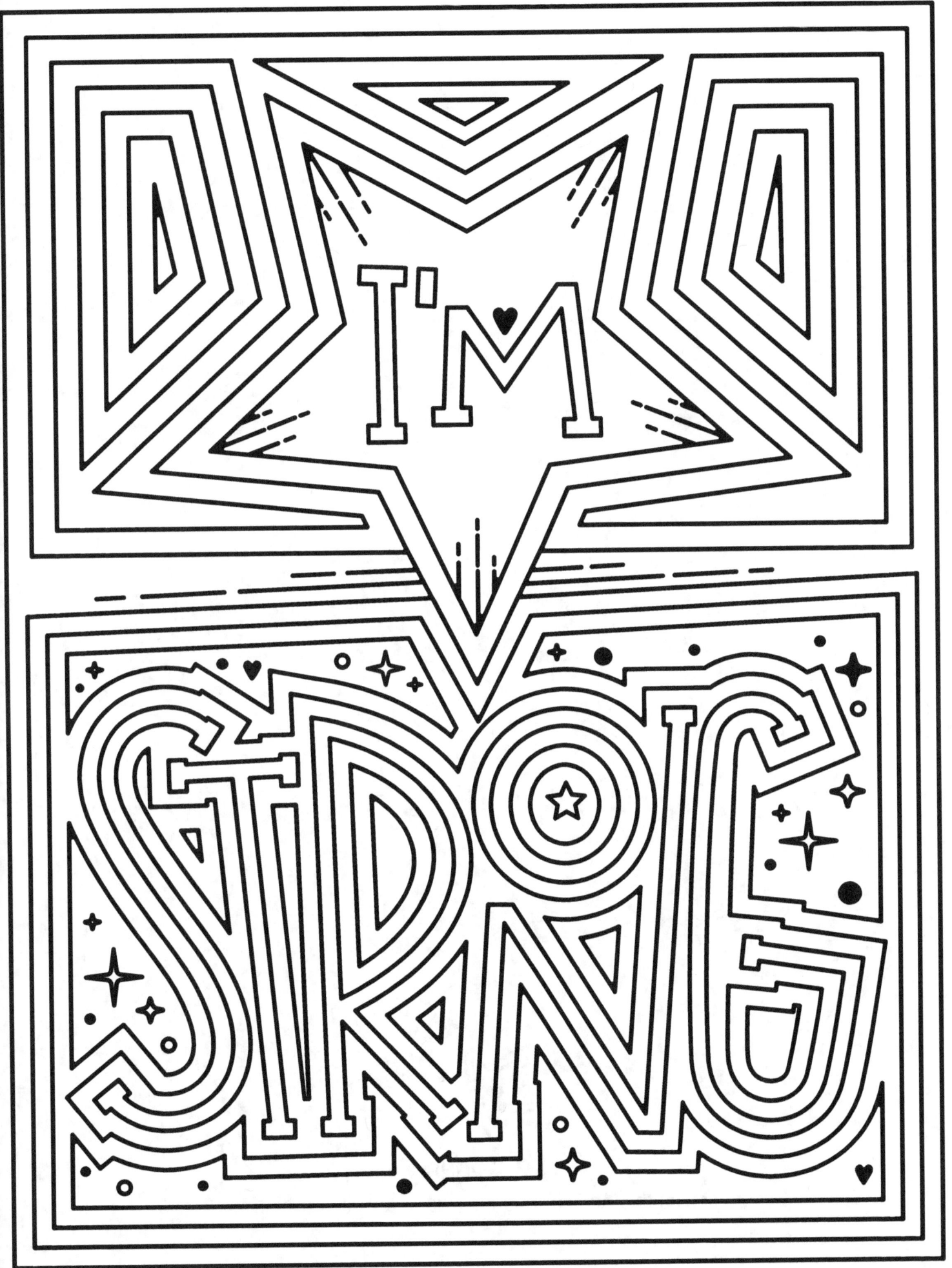

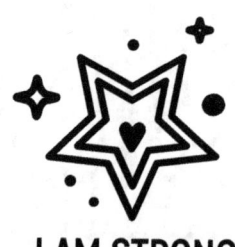

I AM STRONG

I can do this. And I can do this again. You are worth it.

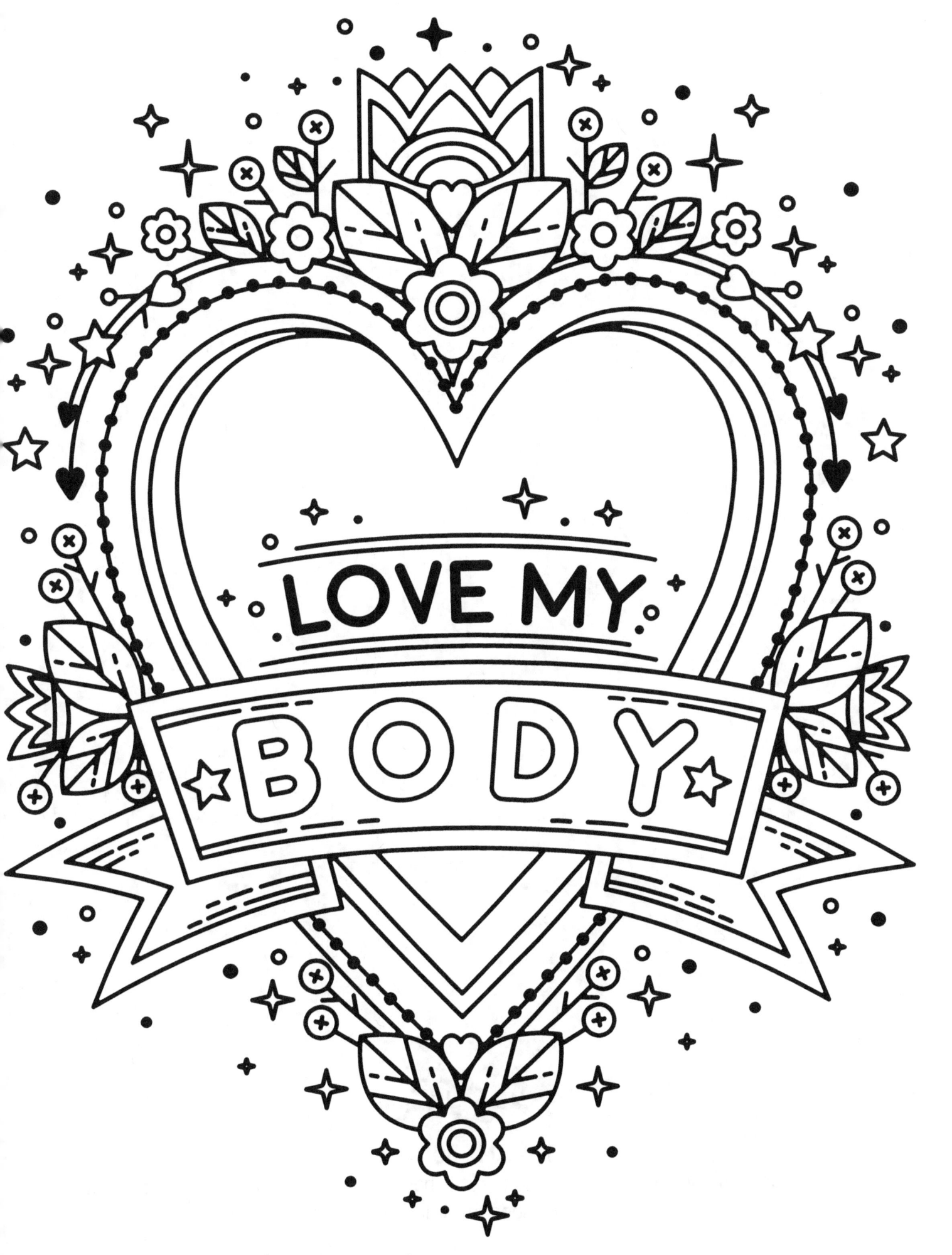

LOVE MY BODY

This body is a great home for you to grow. And I really have the most loving arms to hold you tight.
Come soon my little one.

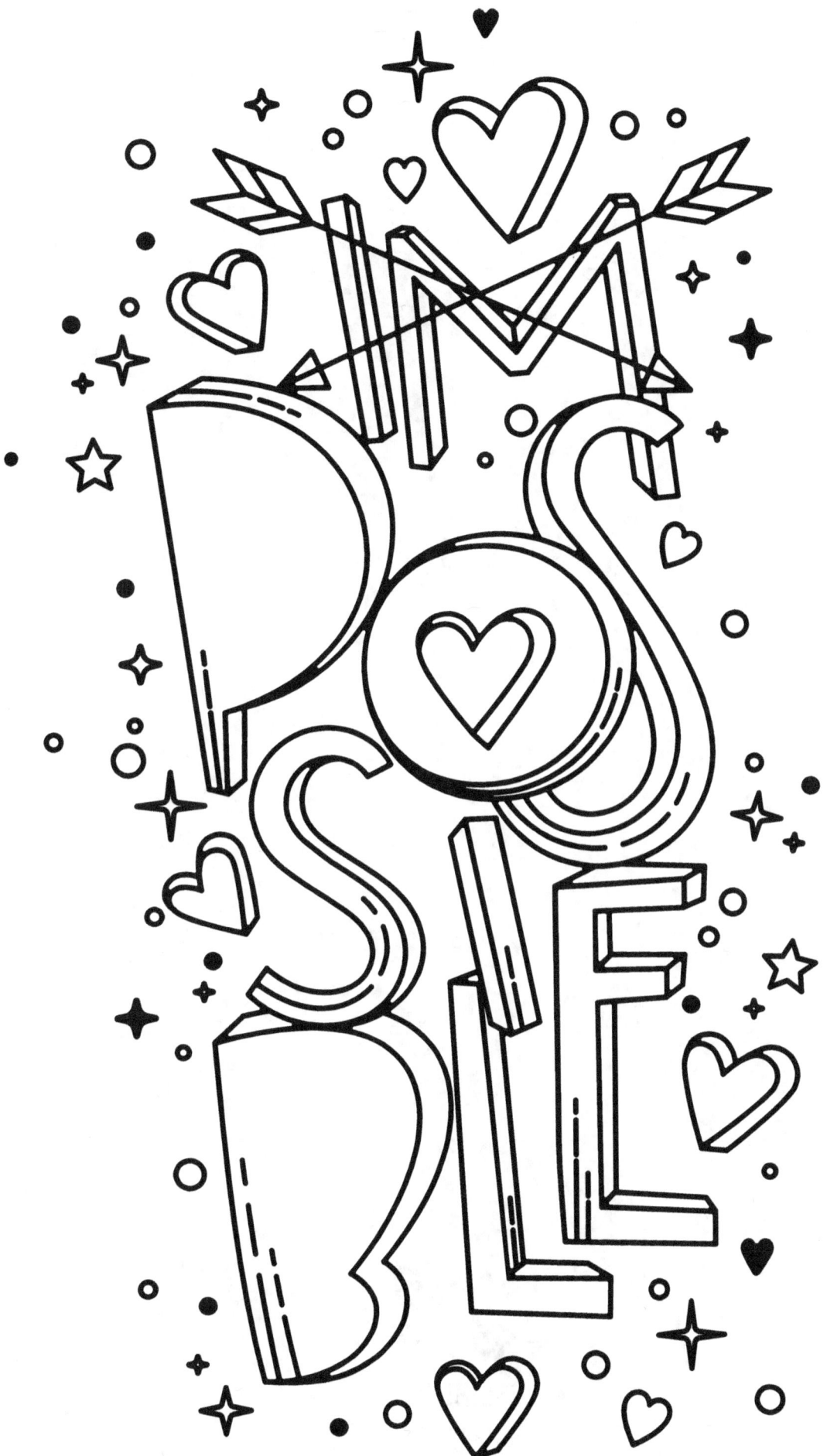

IMPOSSIBLE

Of course we can . We will.

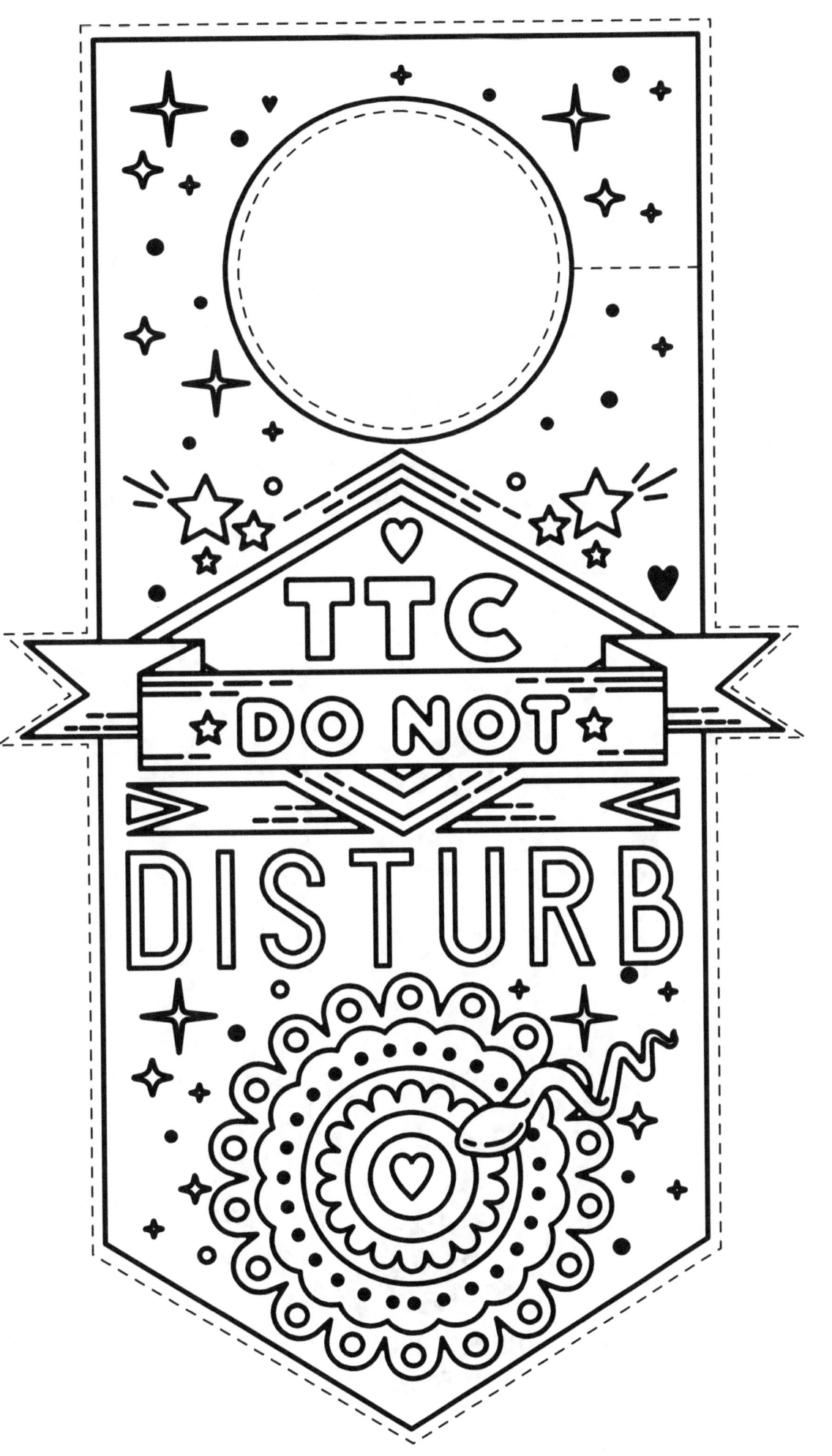

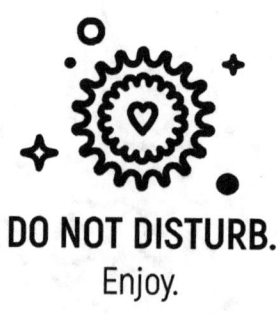

DO NOT DISTURB.

Enjoy.

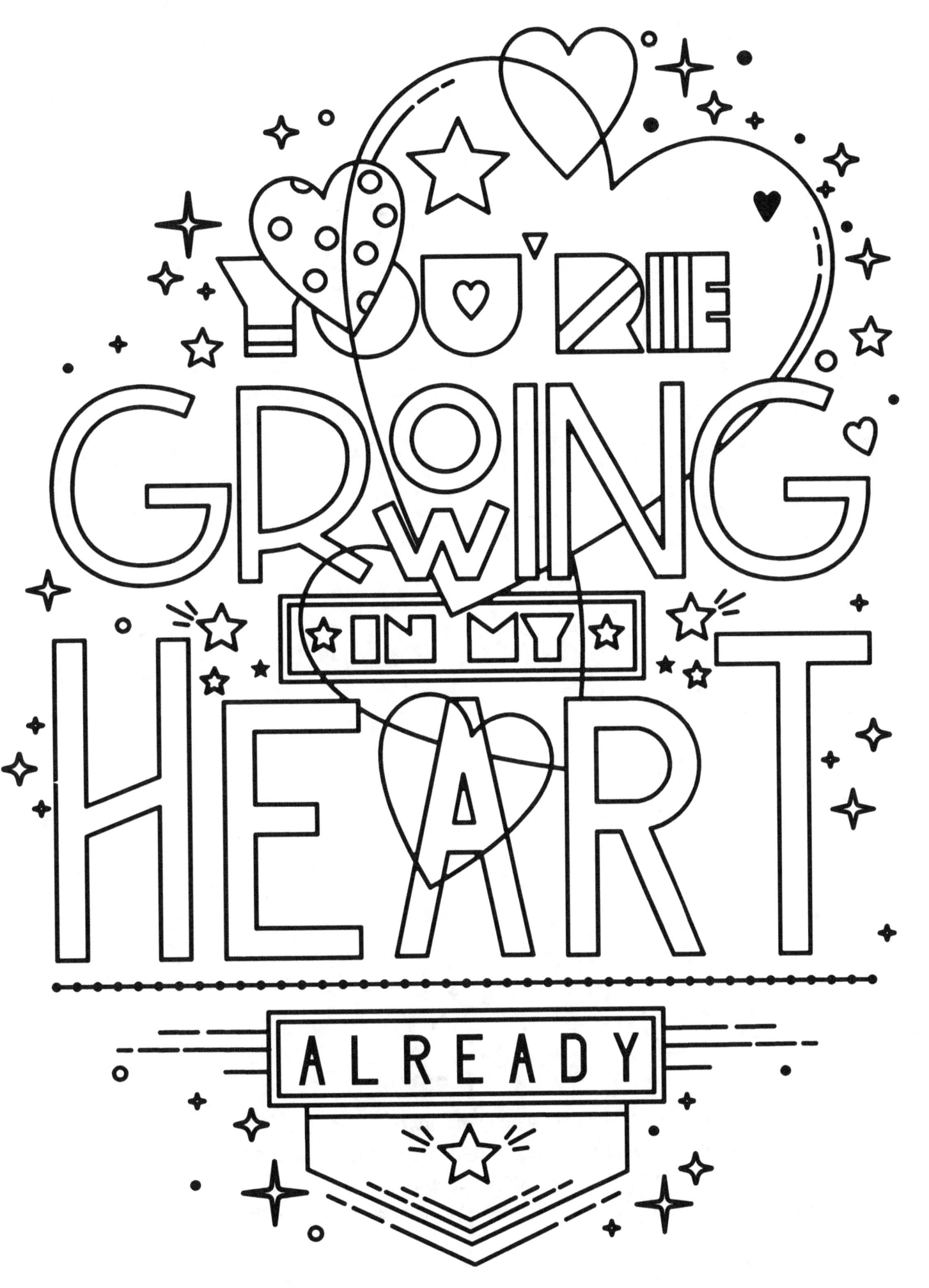

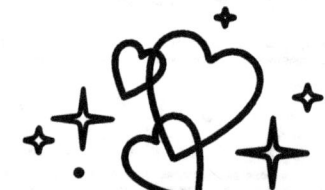

You' re growing in my heart already
I want to be your mom. No matter where or how you are born.
I will be your step, foster, adoptive, but your MOM.
Maybe you're already looking for me and I will keep my eyes open to find you.

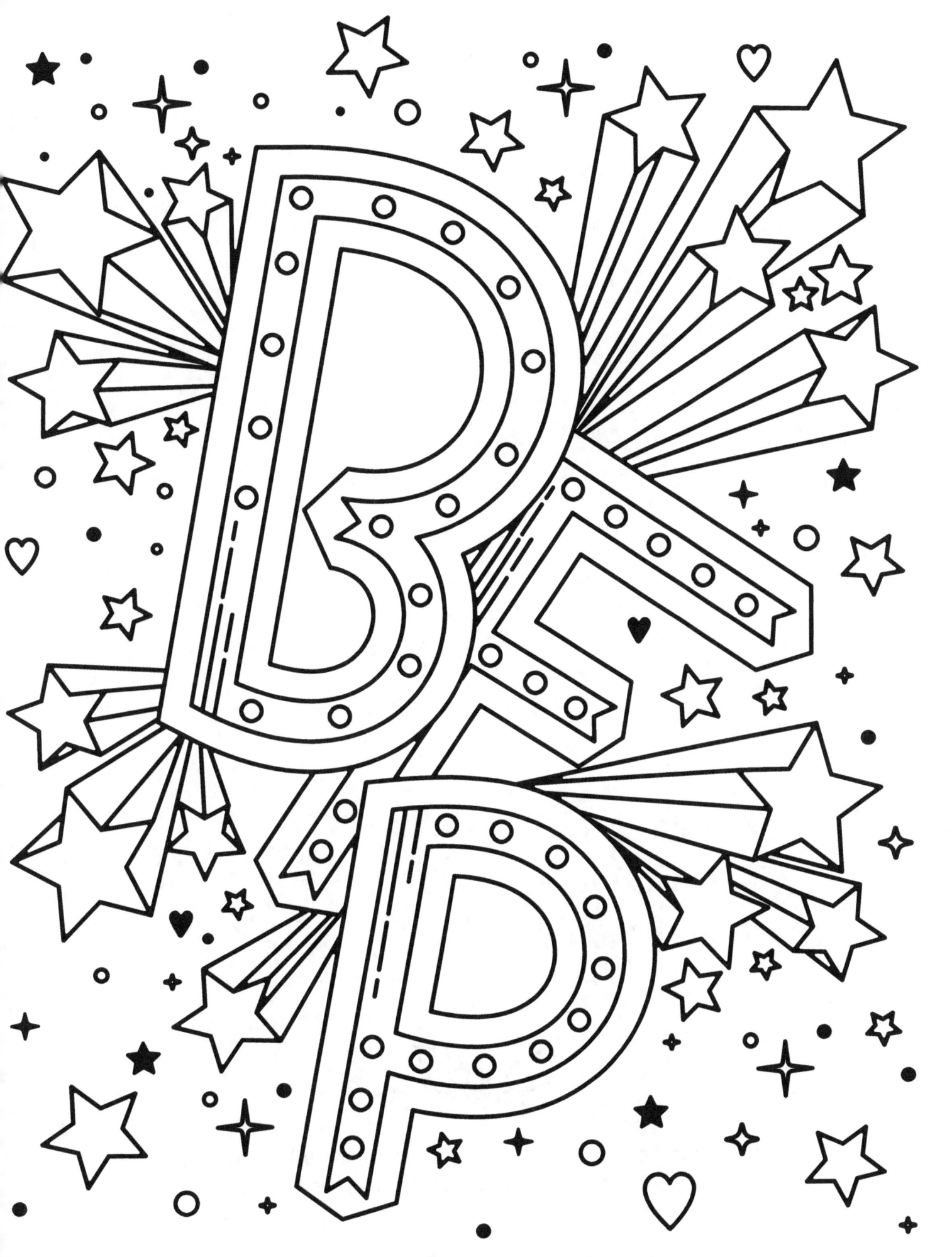

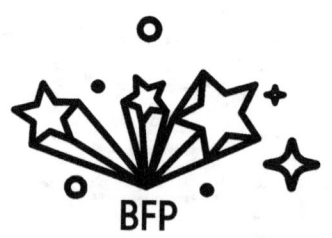

BFP

IWe will BD and then,15 DPO or 2WW, AF wont come, you will be my BFP with
a EDD and me and my DH will forget all this TTC.

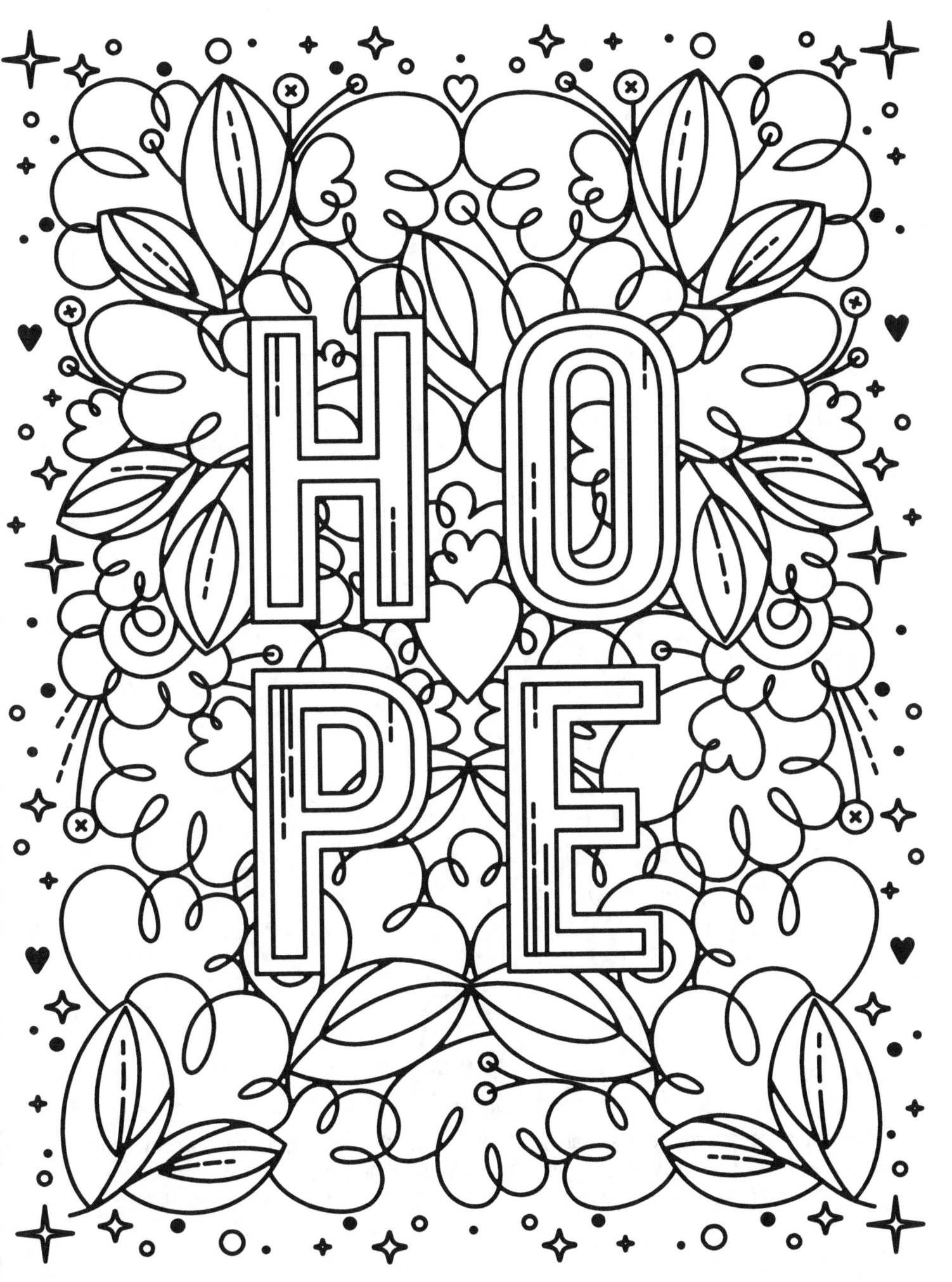

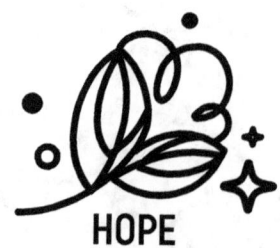

HOPE

Most of the feelings you have now are not beautiful, but they are soooo real: jealousy, anger, dissapointment, loneliness, they are all in you right now. Give them a space, deal with them and mostly, don't blame yourself and between all these, give a big and special place to HOPE.

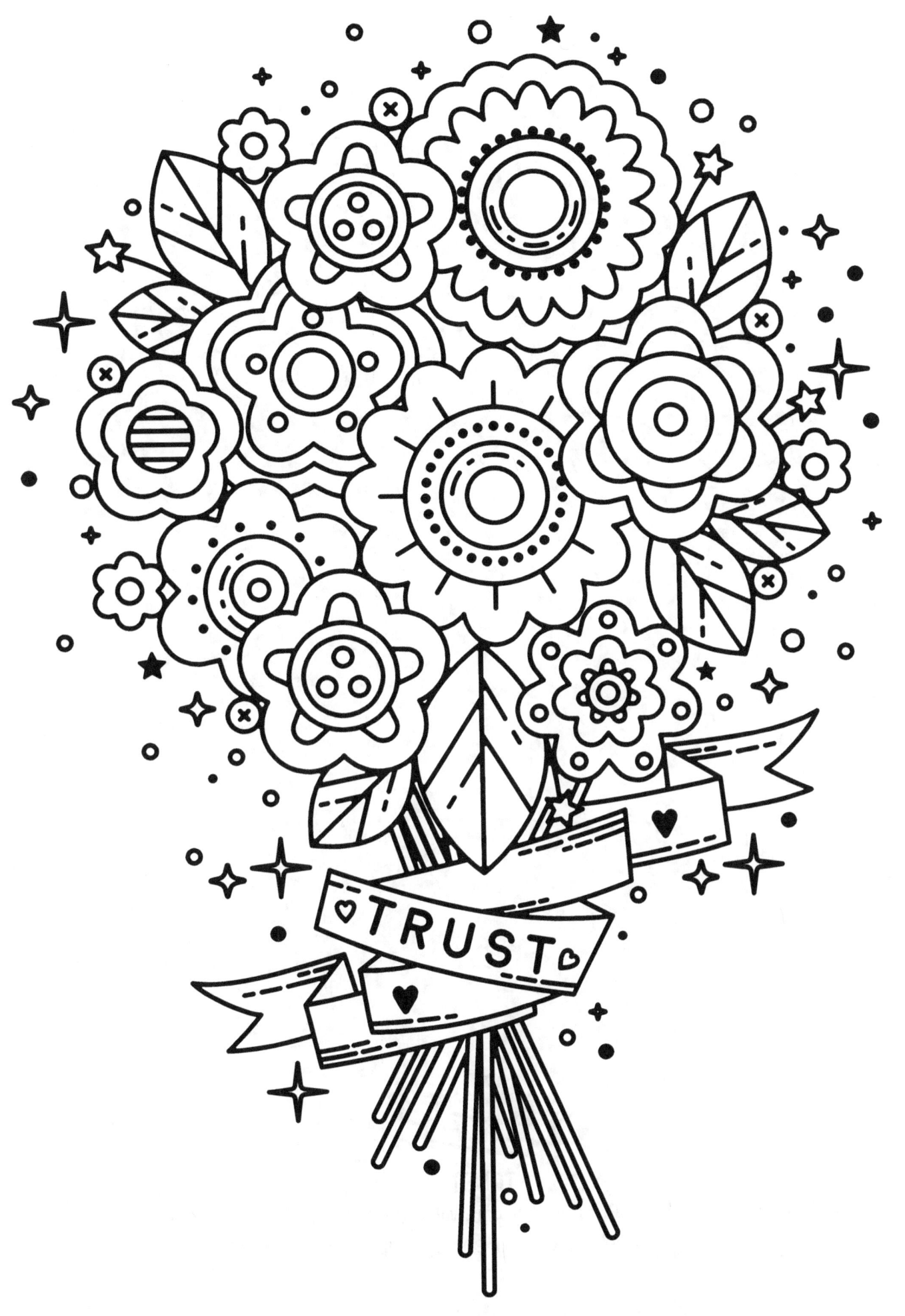

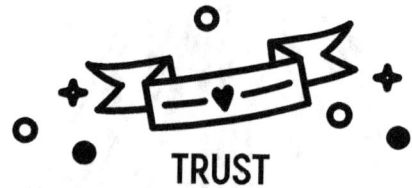

TRUST

Trust your struggle. It's hard. But one day, you will know exactly why it happened this way.
And maybe, one day, you will end up helping someone else.

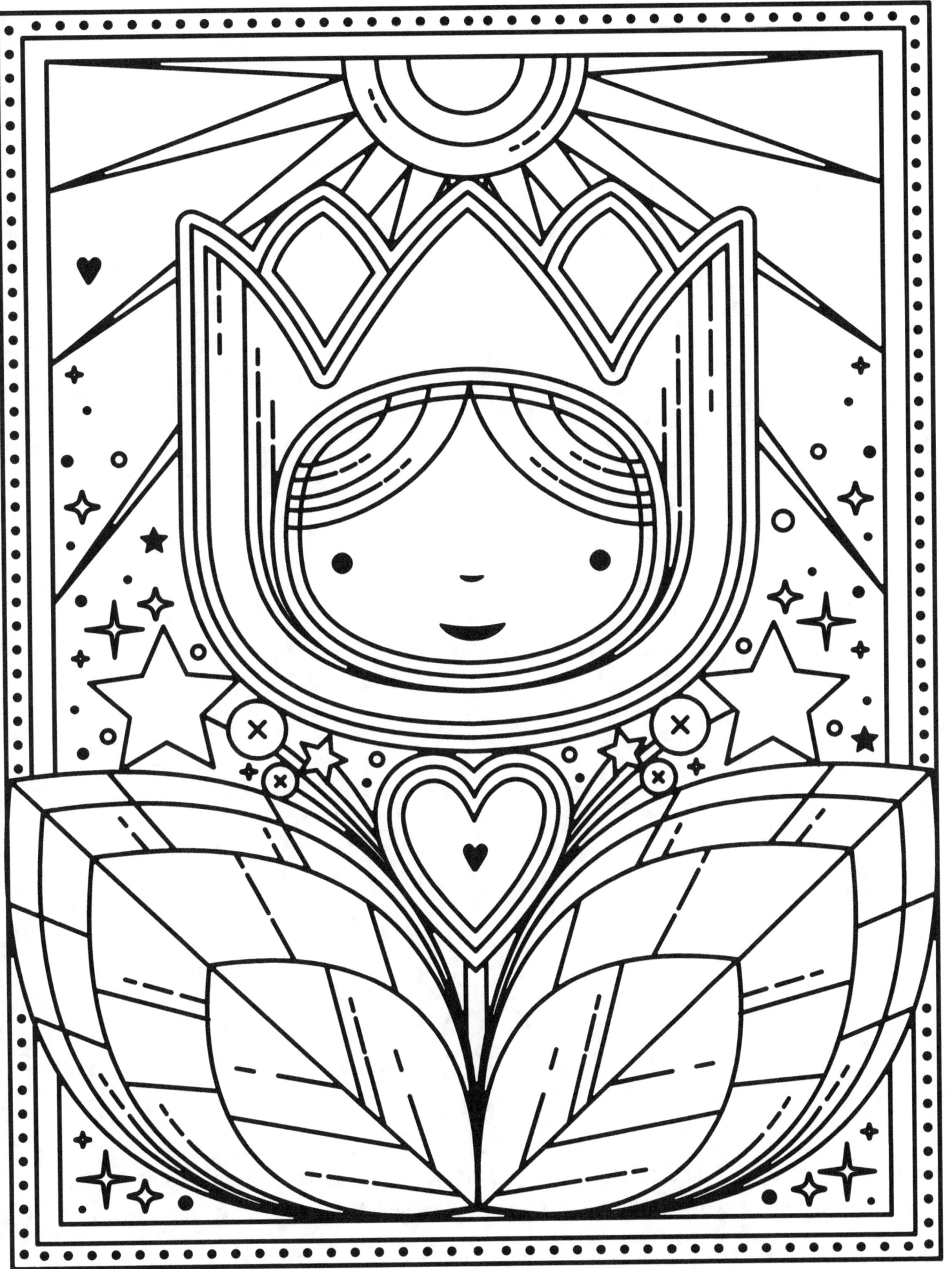

I will keep myself busy doing the things i love and learning new tricks (like a doing a water drop sound with my mouth) to be an amazing and a fun mon! :)